Contents

History and Cultural Significance of Cannabis

Cannabis, also known as marijuana, has a rich history that spans thousands of years and has played a significant role in various cultures around the world. The earliest recorded use of cannabis dates back to ancient civilizations in Asia, where it was primarily used for its medicinal properties. In China, cannabis was mentioned in ancient texts as early as

2700 BCE, and it was revered for its therapeutic effects.

Throughout history, cannabis has been valued for its versatile applications. In ancient India, it was considered a sacred plant and was used in religious ceremonies and meditation practices. In the Middle East, cannabis was cultivated for its fiber, which was used in the production of textiles and ropes. Additionally, cannabis has been used recreationally for its psychoactive properties in many cultures, particularly in regions where it naturally grows.

1.2 Overview of Cannabis Chemistry

Cannabis is a complex plant that contains numerous chemical compounds, which are responsible for its various effects on the human body. The two primary classes of compounds found in cannabis are cannabinoids and terpenes.

Cannabinoids are a diverse group of chemical compounds that interact with the endocannabinoid system (ECS) in the human body. The most well-known cannabinoid is delta-9-tetrahydrocannabinol (THC), which is responsible for the psychoactive effects of cannabis. Another important cannabinoid is cannabidiol (CBD), which has gained significant attention for its potential therapeutic properties without causing intoxication.

Terpenes are aromatic compounds found in many plants, including cannabis. They contribute to the distinct flavors and aromas of different cannabis strains. Terpenes also interact with other compounds, such as cannabinoids, and can influence the overall effects of cannabis. For example, myrcene, a common terpene found in cannabis, is believed to enhance the sedative effects of certain strains.

In addition to cannabinoids and terpenes, cannabis contains other chemical compounds, including flavonoids, phenols, and alkaloids. These compounds contribute to the overall chemical profile of the plant and may have additional therapeutic properties.

1.3 Importance of Cannabis Analysis and Testing

With the increasing popularity and legalization of cannabis for both medical and recreational use, the importance of cannabis analysis and testing has become paramount. Accurate and reliable analysis is crucial for several reasons.

Firstly, cannabis analysis ensures product safety and quality control.

Testing can identify and quantify the levels of cannabinoids, terpenes, and other compounds present in a cannabis product. This information allows consumers to make informed decisions about the products they choose, ensuring that they receive the desired effects and minimizing the risk of adverse reactions.

Secondly, cannabis analysis plays a vital role in regulatory compliance. Many countries and states have implemented regulations and standards for cannabis products to protect consumer safety. These regulations often include testing requirements for contaminants such as pesticides, heavy metals, residual solvents, and microbial contaminants. Analytical testing helps ensure that products meet these regulatory standards and are safe for consumption.

Furthermore, cannabis analysis contributes to scientific research and product development. By understanding the chemical composition of different cannabis strains, researchers can explore the potential therapeutic applications of cannabinoids, terpenes, and other compounds. This knowledge can lead to the development of new medicines and formulations tailored to specific medical conditions.

In conclusion, cannabis chemistry is a fascinating field that encompasses the study of the chemical compounds present in the cannabis plant and their effects on the human body. Understanding the history, cultural significance, and chemical composition of cannabis is crucial in today's rapidly evolving cannabis industry. Accurate analysis and testing of cannabis products ensure safety, quality, and compliance with regulations, while also driving scientific research and innovation in the field of cannabis medicine.

An Introuction To Cannabis Chemistry

Cannabis has been a part of human history for a millennium. Until the early 20th century, it was used as medicine and a spiritual guide in cultures all over the planet.

In the early 1900's it was possible to purchase cannabis tincture at pharmacies, but soon the United States federal government launched a crusade to prohibit this most intriguing plant.

For the last 80 years or so, the major drivers of medical research, pharmaceutical companies, have focused on profitable synthetic drugs and little research has been done on cannabis chemistry and therapeutic applications.

Cannabis Chemistry In Main Stream News

When television personalities like Dr. Oz and Sanjay Gupta are talking about it, it is clear that a wave of change is swelling. Cannabis chemistry contains is much more than a normal plant; it is a gift to humanity with complex scientific secrets.

If you were to walk down the street and ask people what chemicals they associate with marijuana, the overwhelming majority would say THC (and maybe CBD if they saw Dr. Gupta on CNN).

While cannabinoids like THC and CBD are well known and often thought of as the active ingredients in cannabis chemistry, there are a huge number of other chemicals present in the plant.

In order to fully understand the medical applications or to produce quality concentrates or marijuana-infused products, a basic understanding of the science is critical. In addition to the better-known cannabinoids THC and CBD, there are dozens of other related cannabinoids found in the plant's cannabis chemistry.

THCA is the natural product version of THC and understanding the chemistry of these two compounds is of utmost importance. Compounds such as CBC and CBG are chemical precursors in the plant biosynthesis of THC and have been shown to have interesting medical properties.

CBN is a degradation product of THC that has unique physiological effects.

Terpenoids In Cannabis Chemistry

There is also an entire class of compounds called terpenoids that are chemical building blocks to make cannabinoids.

The medical properties of terpenoids are not nearly as well known, but there are certainly some interesting remedies waiting to be discovered in this broad class of chemical compounds.

Cannabinoids and terpenoids are made up of simple chemical building blocks called terpenes.

Terpenes are volatile, small molecules that give cannabis much of its flavor and aroma. They also have unique medical properties and are present in many other plants. Terpenes can be found in pine trees, citrus fruit, and flowers such as lavender and so on.

There is a growing industry across the globe that is focused on using essential oils as therapy for a variety of ailments, so retaining terpenes in concentrates is important for medical reasons. It is also important to understand terpene chemistry as it greatly impacts the texture and flavor of cannabis concentrates.

Compounds In Cannabis Chemistry

In addition to the ever-intriguing cannabinoids, terpenoids, and terpenes, cannabis chemistry also contains a number of other ubiquitous chemical compounds found in many other living things.

Cannabis chemistry contains proteins and enzymes, starches and carbohydrates, waxes and other oils as well as chlorophyll and other common plant chemicals.

While these are not psychoactive and have minimal medical value, it is important to consider these components of cannabis chemistry as well.

They can greatly affect the color, flavor, and texture of concentrates and infused products. Cannabinoids are found throughout virtually the entire cannabis plant at all stages of growth, from seedlings to harvested flowers.

The flowers of the cannabis plant are by far the most potent component in terms of THC and CBD and other cannabinoids in its chemistry. However, the stems and leaves also contain a relatively small amount of cannabinoids.

Cannabis flowers typically test from 10-30% for THC by weight, while leaves and stems are typically 1-5% THC. Each strain of cannabis has a specific cannabinoid profile with THC, CBD, and others present in specific ratios.

While the percent of cannabinoid present in the various parts of the plant will vary, the profile remains pretty much the same for a given strain. Because of recent reports of the medical properties of CBD, there has been significant interest breeding strains with a high CBD content.

Hemp is also a significant source of CBD and other cannabinoids but is subject to different federal and local regulations. Because THC is the primary psychoactive ingredient in cannabis chemistry, it is the most interesting cannabinoid to many people.

A basic understanding of how THC is made in the cannabis plant is essential for anyone who wants to work with cannabis. As mentioned previously, THCA is the natural product formed biosynthetically by cannabis. Unlike THC, THCA is not psychoactive when consumed.

Curing Process In Cannabis Chemistry

During the curing process, THCA in flowers is converted to THC through a process called decarboxylation. This process is also referred to as conversion, activation or decarbing. During decarboxylation, the THCA undergoes a chemical change where it gives off carbon dioxide gas to form THC.

This conversion also takes place when the flowers are heated as they are smoked or vaporized, so even flowers that are not fully decarboxylated will be psychoactive. For edibles and other products that will not be heated prior to ingestion, it is important to know how much THC and THCA are present so that the proper dose can be formulated.

Activating Cannabis Chemistry From THCA To THC

Complete conversion of THCA to THC is simple and can be achieved by heating above 210 °F for extended periods of time.

The plant material can be activated prior to extraction, or the concentrate itself can be decarbed to ensure that all THCA is converted to THC for infused products and this process will be discussed in a subsequent laboratory course.

Cannabinoids, terpenoids, and terpenes are all hydrophobic chemical compounds, meaning they are not very soluble in water but dissolve easily in oils and organic solvents. For this reason, solvents like butane or alcohol are popular methods of extracting cannabis.

It is possible to use water to make bubble hash, but that is a physical separation and not a true extraction where the THC and other plant oils are dissolved in a solvent. The choice of extraction solvent can greatly impact the type and quality of concentrate that will be produced.

Compared to terpenes, cannabinoids have relatively high boiling points above 350 °F while many terpenes boil at less than 200 °F. This difference in boiling point can be used to separate components by distillation in some applications.

It is also important to keep these numbers in mind while purging or decarbing because terpenes may be lost in the process impacting flavor, texture and physiological effects of a concentrate or infused product. THCA and CBD are both solids in their pure form, while THC is thick oil.

Terpenes tend to be thin liquids, although some are crystalline solids at room temperature. The cannabinoids do not only differ in physical and chemical properties as we have just seen, but they also have varying effects on the human body when ingested.

You know that THCA, present in fresh plant material, is not psychoactive and must be heated to convert to THC before consumption to get high.

CBD is not considered to be psychoactive and is actually a cannabinoid receptor antagonist which means that it counters the effects of THC in the brain. However, CBD is claimed to help with pain, inflammation, seizures, mental illness and many other ailments so there is much demand for it, even though it does not induce a high.

CBN is a degradation product of THC and is known to cause drowsiness when ingested. Other, lesser-known cannabinoids like CBC and CBG have not been studied as well. As the science around cannabis chemistry advances, there will be more and more clinical studies to determine how natural and synthetic cannabinoids affect our bodies and minds.

You should now have a basic understanding of the broad classes of chemicals that are found in cannabis chemistry, their physical and chemical chemistry properties and how they affect users.

Let us know what you think.

Cannabis Concentrates and Infused Products

For many years the primary method of consumption for marijuana in modern society has been smoking the flowers which contain most of the THC and other cannabinoids found in the plant.

Sure, some people like to bake infused brownies and others use vaporizers, but the vast majority prefers to pack a bowl or light a joint. That is rapidly changing as medical marijuana is becoming increasingly legal in the U.S. and other countries.

Hashish, or hash, has been around since ancient times and is a concentrated form of cannabis that is popular as an alternative to smoking cannabis flowers. In this blog, we will explore the many different types of cannabis concentrates, the various methods of making them and how they can be consumed or used to make infused products.

Whether you call it BHO, hash, honey oil, Tears of Phoenix, an extraction or cannabis concentrates, there are a thriving culture and significant amount of science behind this wonderful goo. For as long as human beings have known about the cannabis plant, we have been experimenting with methods to obtain higher doses of the main psychoactive ingredient, THC.

Simple methods employ mechanical and physical separation of the resin-rich glands that contain most of the active ingredients to produce a rather crude cannabis concentrate that has a lower potency and a high amount of plant material.

20th Century Cannabis Concentrates

In the 20th century, chemical extraction became increasingly popular with books like Cannabis Alchemy by D. Gold explaining how solvents such as alcohol or petroleum-based hydrocarbons can be used to produce very potent and pure cannabis concentrates.

Not long thereafter, butane honey oil or BHO as it is often called became popular because it can be produced easily and quickly with cheap and readily available materials.

In the new millennium, cannabis concentrates got a high tech boost as super-critical carbon dioxide extraction, the same process used to make decaf coffee, began being used to make hash. Now there are a handful of companies that produce extractors that are designed specifically for making hash, although many are marketed as generic herbal essential oil extractors for legal reasons.

The earliest hashish was not surprisingly the simplest form of cannabis concentrate. The buds of the cannabis plant are covered in tiny glands called trichomes, which can be thought of as cannabinoid factories where the plant makes most of its THC and other similar compounds.

When the flowers are rubbed or otherwise mechanically agitated, the trichomes separate from the plant material and bring along a lot of cannabinoids with them. For example, when cannabis flowers are being harvested and manicured a significant amount of resin becomes stuck to the scissors being used to trim the plants.

This sticky, dark solid is often referred to as "scissor hash" and is usually a cultivator's first opportunity to sample some of their new harvests. Ancient people in Western Asia prepared crude hashish using similar methods to remove trichomes from the plant material to make some of the first cannabis concentrates in the world.

A simple modification to this basic procedure produces a higher quality hash that has been termed "bubble hash". By using water to aid in the separation of the resin glands from the rest of the plant material, a much lighter colored and higher potency hash can be obtained.

The water helps to remove chlorophyll and other impurities from the hash, thus resulting in lighter colored oil with a higher THC potency. While bubble hash made with water is a concentrated form of cannabis, it is physical separation and not a true extract.

Solvent Extraction To Make Cannabis Concentrates

Extraction is a process that involves the use of a solvent to dissolve the essential oils in the plant and chemically separate them from the plant material, not all that different from making tea or coffee. There are many advantages to extracting cannabis with a solvent, the greatest being the ability to filter the extract and remove all of the plant material.

This will afford a cannabis concentrate that is more potent, burns/vaporizes cleaner and is easier to infuse into products such as edibles or vaporizer pens. Using a liquid solvent also allows the extract to be refined and purified to remove color, waxes and other impurities.

Using extraction methods, it is possible to obtain cannabis extracts that are upwards of 90% THC. There are, however, some drawbacks to using certain extraction solvents that can have major health and safety implications which will be discussed in more detail later.

Simple Fat-Based Cannabis Concentrates

The simplest cannabis extracts are fat-based cannabis concentrates such as infused butter or cooking oils like canola, coconut or olive oil. The fat-based concentrates are prepared by steeping cannabis plant material in the fat while heating to extract cannabinoids and other phytochemicals.

The plant material is then strained and the fat-based cannabis concentrate is ready for oral consumption. Often these cannabis concentrates are used to make infused edible products like candies and baked goods.

Whenever a fat-based cannabis concentrate is to be eaten, it is important to activate the plant material prior to extraction. Activation is the process that converts the non-psychoactive, natural product THCA to its psychoactive form, THC.

This decarboxylation reaction can be achieved by heating the plant material above 210 degrees Fahrenheit for at least an hour. Although glycerin is not technically a fat, it can be used to prepare a tincture in a similar manner as with cooking oils.

Because fat-based and glycerin cannabis concentrates are prepared by direct infusion of plant material into the fat, the THC potency of the oil is unknown. The infused fat must be tested for potency before it can be used to make precision dosed products.

Alternatively, hash that is made from solvent extraction and tested for potency can be diluted with a known amount of fat to prepare an infusion of known potency. The vast majority of commercial marijuana-infused products manufacturers use this method, while direct infusion is generally used by individuals at home.

One major drawback of the fat-based cannabis concentrates is that it is very difficult, if not impossible, to isolate the THC and other cannabinoids from the cooking oil to make hash. Cooking oils are not volatile, meaning they have a high boiling point and cannot be removed by distillation.

Cannabis Concentrates Using Volatile Solvents

a volatile solvent is used in place of the cooking oil, it can be distilled off resulting in a high potency hash. When using volatile solvents to extract cannabis, it is important to fully remove or purge all of the solvents from the hash for health and safety reasons.

This is usually done with a vacuum chamber and/or heat to boiling off the residual solvent. There are a number of volatile organic solvents that are used to extract cannabis, but butane is by far the most popular.

Butane is cheap and readily available and also has a very low boiling point of 30 degrees Fahrenheit, so it is simple to purge the solvent from the concentrate. Butane is used by home and commercial producers alike to make very high-quality hash but has some serious safety risks.

Butane is a highly flammable compressed gas, so extractions using butane should be done outside or in a well-ventilated room with a spark-free exhaust fan to prevent explosions. The use of butane to extract cannabis is illegal in many areas, so it is important to know the law before blasting your own hash.

The toxicity of butane is low, but it is still important to purge all of the butane from the hash and this must also be done safely and responsibly. Most people make BHO by "open-blasting" where they force compressed butane through a tube or column containing the plant material and collect the hash in a pan and the end of the tube.

This process is dangerous, wastes butane and also sends butane into the atmosphere where it can have a negative environmental impact. Some states have banned open blasting for commercial hash production and require the use of expensive recapture machines that recycle almost all of the butane.

Other Volatile Organic Solvents

An alternative to butane blasting is the use of other volatile organic solvents with higher boiling points to extract hash. Grain alcohol such as Everclear (95% ethanol) or hexane is common liquid extraction solvents with respective boiling points of 173 and 154 degrees Fahrenheit.

Other common solvents include petroleum ether, isopropyl alcohol, acetone or liquid hydrocarbons such as pentane or heptane. The choice of solvent will greatly impact the quality of the cannabis concentrate and we will go into more detail on this in a subsequent blog focused on the solvent extraction of cannabis.

Non-polar solvents such as hexane are quite selective for cannabinoids and other essential oils in the plant and give a high purity and potency hash. More polar solvents like alcohols or acetone are less selective and will extract chlorophyll and other phytochemicals resulting in a darker, less pure and less potent hash.

Because the boiling points of these solvents are higher, they are liquids at room temperature which allows for simple and direct chemical manipulation of the cannabis concentrates. While the hash is still dissolved in the solvent, it can be purified to remove colors or waxes to give a more potent or cleaner hash and this is not possible with butane.

Many of the liquid solvents used to extract cannabis such as hexane or isopropyl alcohol are toxic, so it is critical to purge all of the solvents from the hash and test for residual solvent using gas chromatography. The only liquid solvent that is considered safe and is acceptable to have residual solvent in the hash is ethanol because it has very low toxicity.

Super-Critical Carbon Dioxide Extraction

Another extraction method that is becoming increasingly popular to prepare hash is super-critical carbon dioxide extraction. This process is used industrially to produce decaffeinated coffee and to extract essential oils for flavorings and fragrances.

The carbon dioxide is compressed in a chamber until it reaches the super-critical phase which is a hybrid liquid-gas. Under these conditions, the CO_2 can act as a solvent and will dissolve organic material such as cannabinoids.

Because there are no organic solvents used in the process, it is usually thought of as the cleanest extraction method for making hash. If that's the case, then you may wonder why people are still using butane and liquid organic solvents.

That is because super-critical CO2 extractors are expensive and range from about $20,000 all the way up to $250,000. Additionally, the operation of these machines is complex and requires a highly skilled operator.

To obtain high yields and good quality hash with this process is not trivial, the maintenance and repairs of this type of extractor can also be costly. A handful of extraction artists are able to make great quality hash with carbon dioxide extraction, but much of the time the hash oil that is obtained is a thin, runny consistency and will be used in edibles or vaporizer pen formulas.

Cannabis Concentrates Final Points

There is a wide range of textures of cannabis concentrates that can be made. The properties of the final product are highly dependent upon the starting plant material, the extraction process and post-extraction processing and refinement.

Bubble hash made by water extraction is typically solid with a dark amber to brown to green color. Hash oil made by extraction with butane or liquid solvents can have a wide range of textures from very thin and runny honey oil, to thicker sap-like consistency to the much-coveted shatter.

The viscosity of the hash oil is highly dependent upon the terpene content of the oil. Terpenes are low molecular weight, volatile oils that are responsible for the flavor and aroma of cannabis.

By purging the hash oil in a vacuum oven at elevated temperatures, many of the terpenes are evaporated off leaving very high potency oil that has a crystalline structure that is known as shatter.

The wax content of the hash will also impact its texture so strains that are very rich in paraffin waxes tend to yield the hash oil that is more opaque and softer, earning names such as butter or earwax.

Waxes can be removed through a process called winterization which we will cover in detail later in this series of blogs. Cannabis concentrates can be used in many ways for recreational and medicinal purposes, they can be added to the cooking oil in a recipe and used to make infused edible products of all sorts.

It is also possible to make gel capsules with precise doses of THC, CBD or other cannabinoids. Cannabis concentrates can be smoked on their own, or people often combine them with cannabis flower when smoking.

In recent years, dabbing has become very popular for cannabis concentrates. To do a dab, a piece of metal or glass is heated with a torch and concentrate is applied and immediately vaporizes and is inhaled.

There are also tabletop and portable electronic vaporizers that work in a similar manner by heating an electric coil. Electronic cigarette vaporizers that are the size of an ink pen are becoming hugely popular, some of the vape pens work with pure concentrate, while others require it to be thinned with some sort of carrier such as glycerin.

This blog was intended to introduce the various types of cannabis concentrates and methods that are used to make them. As you can see, this is a complex topic that is closely related to the chemistry of the cannabis plant.